FINALLY!!! STOP HAVING COLDS & FLU

PHARMACIST J. ALBERT HERMLE

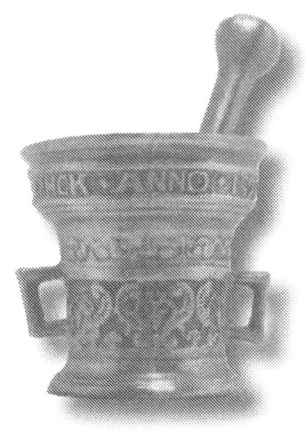

Order this book online at www.trafford.com/07-0249
or email orders@trafford.com

Most Trafford titles are also available at major online book retailers.

Note for Librarians: A cataloguing record for this book is available from Library and Archives Canada at www.collectionscanada.ca/amicus/index-e.html

ISBN: 978-1-4251-1839-6

THE COVER:

Pictured is a sixteenth century Dutch Pharmacy Mortar & Pestle cast in a Foundry at Deventer, the Netherlands, CIRCA 1590.

We at Trafford believe that it is the responsibility of us all, as both individuals and corporations, to make choices that are environmentally and socially sound. You, in turn, are supporting this responsible conduct each time you purchase a Trafford book, or make use of our publishing services. To find out how you are helping, please visit www.trafford.com/responsiblepublishing.html

Our mission is to efficiently provide the world's finest, most comprehensive book publishing service, enabling every author to experience success. To find out how to publish your book, your way, and have it available worldwide, visit us online at www.trafford.com/10510

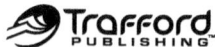 www.trafford.com

North America & international
toll-free: 1 888 232 4444 (USA & Canada)
phone: 250 383 6864 ♦ fax: 250 383 6804 ♦ email: info@trafford.com

The United Kingdom & Europe
phone: +44 (0)1865 722 113 ♦ local rate: 0845 230 9601
facsimile: +44 (0)1865 722 868 ♦ email: info.uk@trafford.com

10 9 8 7 6 5 4

THANK YOU
to
Lynden Gellner
Joan Hermle
&
Jill Terry
for their assistance in the
publication of this book

And A VERY SPECIAL THANK YOU to all my many
prescription patients, pharmacy customers, and
friends who over the years provided feedback and
answered numerous questions about their health in
my search for a cure for the "common cold"

"YOU ALL ASSISTED IN MAKING THIS BOOK POSSIBLE"

A SPECIAL ACKNOWLEDGMENT
AND
THANK YOU
TO
PHARMACIST

ARTHUR HARASEK

MY PHARMACY MENTOR

"If anyone ever discovers a cure for the common cold, he or she will be a shoo-in for the Nobel Prize."

Time magazine, October 13, 1987

According to a recent National Academy of Science study,
a new pandemic, which is a WIDE SPREAD epidemic,
of the influenza virus is not only inevitable, but is long over due.
Since there are currently no known cures for the COMMON cold
and flu, prevention must be everyone's goal!

J. Albert

Contents

FINALLY!!!
STOP HAVING
COLDS & FLU

DEDICATED TO
Sophie Jusick
&
Arlette Billings

JUST WHO ARE Sophie Jusick and Arlette Billings that *FINALLY!!! STOP HAVING COLDS & FLU* is dedicated?

Sophie Jusick . . .

Sophie was my grandmother, my mother's mother. She was a grandmother I never got to know. She died about 13 years before I was born from complications brought on by a bout of the flu during the great pandemic of the Spanish Flu during 1918–1920. In this time frame, it is estimated between 50 and 100 million people died as victims of this infectious disease. MORE PEOPLE DIED AS RESULT OF COMING DOWN WITH THE FLU THAN ALL THE PEOPLE KILLED IN BATTLE DURING WORLD WAR I.

Arlette Billings . . .

Arlette was a very outgoing, fun loving, caring family oriented person. Her husband passed away a few years before she sold the multimillion dollar family business that they worked very hard to build. She had many loving friends and relatives and a beautiful new home in St. Charles, Illinois. She was ready to relax and enjoy the "good life." At the age of 58 she died in the middle of the summer of complications brought on by the "common cold." Arlette was my cousin. Sophie Jusick was also Arlette's grandmother.

Preface

MOST OF THE material presented in *Finally!!! Stop Having Colds & FLU* is very different from what you'll discover in most health publications. What's different? Well, you'll find no index or bibliography. Presented in this publication are my own recollections and documentations about the "common cold" and flu. The presentation of the information I reveal to you will be as if you were a prescription patient or customer in a pharmacy where I was practicing.

Presented here are my personal recollections and documentations of colds and flu, which are a result of over 50 years of personal observations as a retail pharmacist . . . over 50 years of my own research, reading countless numbers of news articles, magazine publications, medical bulletins, health newsletters, pharmaceutical brochures and attending health related seminars . . . and most important my over 50 years of personal experimentation pertaining to viruses and bacteria that bring on bouts of colds, flu, and "head colds" that people are forced to endure. You will find some references to information I present that I have documented. Only what I consider the important references will be listed right along with the text. Very seldom as a practicing pharmacist while giving a health recommendation to patients did I announce my source of the information and/or from what page the health info came. On completion of this book I discarded two full 37 gallon plastic garbage sacks containing newspaper articles, health magazines, and all sort of clippings pertaining to colds and flu.

As stated above, I am going to present information to you as if you were a patient or customer in a pharmacy or drugstore –as if I was serving you. You'll notice while reading this book there are many what I hope you'll find short humorous anecdotal stories, jokes, health facts, and personal comments I elude to, to help present my findings on colds and flu. Many are the same stories I told my pharmacy patients while delivering them their prescription medications. The stories are called "SIDELITES" in this book. I find a little humor along with informational health discoveries goes along way in getting health messages across to people. Some of my pharmacy patients mentioned listening to me was like listening to an entertaining health advertisement or commercial. At the end of this book I have some "Outtakes." I hope you'll enjoy them. *Many who have followed my advice on various health-related issues over the years have maintained happy, healthier lives. How do I know? They told me so.*

My approach to health for the public and myself has always been that of "prevention." Find the cause of ill health and eliminate it to stay healthy for now and in the future. As it has been said in sports, and I'm sure you've heard it said many times, "The best offense is the good defense." Remember, in life diseases are everyone's most formidable opponent!

Although my profession was the dispensing of pills, I've always professed that the fewer pills and medicines one takes the better. However, during times of need pills and medicines should be used according to your doctor's instructions. It is my belief that everyone must supplement their diet with a daily vitamin preparation. The vitamins are a "form of dietary insurance" to maintain better health. Many times on days when there was a slowdown in the prescription business in the pharmacies where I practiced, the pharmacy technicians most often jokingly scolded me by telling me that I told too many people how to stay healthy, and that's why we weren't filling many prescriptions that day.

Again I repeat, my philosophy has and always will be, *STAY HEALTHY SO YOU DON'T HAVE TO "TAKE PILLS FOR YOUR ILLS."* Each day you are ill is like losing a day in your life. There's a law in physics that states; "for every action there is an opposite and equal reaction." To apply this law to an individual's health, I have always thought that for each day you're ill, the equal and opposite reaction is one day less at the end of your life, yet alone the miserable day spent being sick. Conversely, for every day a person in any manner works to improve their health, a day is added to their life.

As a pharmacist, prevention of illness has always been my greatest interest. It's interesting to note that while spending years of searching for a cure to the common cold, instead I discovered NOT a cure, but a way to prevent it.

I want you to know that I do not consider myself a "guru" in the matters of preventive health... I'M JUST AN OBSERVER OF NATURE AND ITS PREVENTIVE HEALTH POWERS.

Also, I don't consider myself a writer; however, I decided to write "Finally!!! Stop Having Colds & Flu" to get the word out and reveal my preventive antiviral discovery for all. I've always cared for and was concerned about the health of all my pharmacy patients thoughout the years I practiced pharmacy. And now as the reader of this book, I care for you.

Can the information revealed in this book prevent a world wide flu pandemic? Only time will tell.

SPECIAL NOTE...I believe that if many of today's health presentations were given in a more entertaining and/or humorous manner, more of these important messages would be paid greater attention and followed to give many more people an opportunity to lead a longer and healthier life.

MULTIVITAMIN/MULTIMINERAL SUPPLEMENT
SPECIAL NOTICE
Like most people do and I have done throughout
FINALLY!!! STOP HAVING COLDS & FLU, when I
allude to a vitamin or vitamins, I'm referring to a
vitamin and mineral containing product...
a MULTIVITAMIN/MULTIMINERAL SUPPLEMENT.
Proper balances of minerals, like vitamins, are also
essential for insurance of a healthy diet.

"Good health is an asset many do not value until they lose it, and after once lost too often not all the money in the world can buy it back."

—J. ALBERT
  1930 - 20??

"There is a wisdom in this beyond the rules of physic: a man's own observation, what he finds good of, and what he feels hurt of, is the best physic to preserve health."

—Sir Francis Bacon
  1561–1626

THE BEGINNING

It was a typical January morning in Seattle . . . not too cold, but dark and raining at 5:30 AM as I stepped outside on the front porch to retrieve my morning edition of the *Seattle Times* newspaper. I came inside, turned on my coffeemaker for my morning cups of coffee and sat down at the kitchen table to scan the first section of the paper. Almost immediately a news article caught my eye.

"FLU GETS DEADLIER AS NATION GETS OLDER"

"Hey!" I said to myself. "That's me!" I'm 72 years old, and I'll be 73 in July.

The news article related the fact that the National Centers for Disease Control concluded deaths caused by influenza have increased to nearly twice as many as researchers previously believed. The annual toll has climbed from 20,000 deaths a year in the 1970's to an average of 36,000 a year in the 1990's—with the number of deaths soaring to a high of 70,000 in some years. This is according to a study in the *Journal of the American Medical Association.*

The article went on to state that about 90% of all deaths occur among people over 65, and those over 80 are 32 times as likely to die from side effects of the flu as those between the ages of 60 and 65. And as the population of elderly people continues to grow, simple demographics almost ensure a disastrous increase in deaths of this group.

After reading this news article, I felt it was time to write this book. Also, I was almost 3 years into my retirement, and I personally felt it was time to utilize this free time and let the world know of my antiviral find.

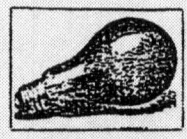

SIDE LITE

It seems like the further I get into retirement the longer it takes me to accomplish almost absolutely nothing.

That's right, it was time to utilize and pass on my personal observations, research, and experimentation on colds and flu.

It was in 1977 that a portion of the prevention method for colds and flu was realized. In 1982 another startling revelation combined with the 1977 discovery gave credence to my cold and flu prevention method . . . A METHOD SO NATURAL, SIMPLE, AND EASY TO DO. IT'S UNBELIEVABLE!! I will reveal this method to you later in *J. Albert Antiviral Report*. Along with this method, I will refer to the sources of information which led me to this long sought after amazing discovery.

It's been reported in the U.S. alone that over 40 billion dollars a year is spent by the American public on cold and flu related items. This dollar number includes the cost of lost wages, doctor visits, and medication costs. And there's no tally on the misery and suffering that the colds and flu can cause. Now where did I get the 40 billion dollar figure? It was taken from a drug company poster in my doctor's examination room while I was waiting for my yearly physical. Again, I saw the same 40 billion dollar number in several news articles on colds and flu.

Read on and discover my natural, easy to follow method to make the common cold and flu uncommon to you, your family, and with all those who you share this health information.

All About J. Albert

ONE COULD SAY that the discovery that led to the publication of *FINALLY!!! STOP HAVING COLDS & FLU* began just over 58 years ago. It started in the middle of June 1944 in the city of Berwyn, Illinois, a southwest suburb of Chicago. The world was in the throes of World War II, and I had just graduated eighth grade from the John J. Pershing grammar school and in the fall preparing to enter Fenwick Highschool in Oak Park.

In those days the local drugstore was the focal point and meeting place of the neighborhood. It was a time before mass retail marketing. Drugstores sold mainly drugs, grocery stores sold groceries, gas stations were called service stations and sold only gas and oil. However, it was common for the corner drugstore to have an ice cream soda fountain. Outside of previously delivering the *Downtown Shopping News* advertising newspaper—315 newspapers for pay of 90¢ to $1.10 depending on the number of pages in the paper—it was the local corner drugstore soda fountain that provided me with what I considered my first real employment - that of a dream position of "soda jerk." I was in ice cream heaven making ice cream sundaes, sodas, and milk shakes at the price of 20¢ each. Along with the soda fountain duties I was responsible for the sales of penny candy and 5 cent candy bars from a case next to the soda fountain. That's right - candy bars were 5¢ each, and for the price of 10¢ you could purchase a quarter pound size Baby Ruth® candy bar. There were times when Art, the candy salesman, would deliver Baby Ruth® candy bars to the drugstore, and the bars were still warm coming right from the old Curtiss Candy factory.

My dream position at the drugstore paid 25¢ an hour plus, and now get this, all the soda fountain goodies and candy I could eat while on duty. I gained 20 pounds in my first six months on the job.

VonDraseks Pharmacy was the name of the corner drugstore, and it was located on the corner of Ogden and Ridgeland in Berwyn about 9 miles southwest of Downtown Chicago on old Route 66. The drugstore was just four blocks from where I grew up. Three pharmacist brothers owned and operated the store. The older two brothers, Otto and Joe, graduated from pharmacy school at the University of Notre Dame. While they attended the school, Knute Rockne was its legendary football coach. John, the youngest brother was a University of Illinois pharmacy graduate.

One spring Joe and his young nephew departed on a tour of the northwest United States. While on the last leg of their tour, Joe, who was diabetic, died of complications brought on by the disease. His unfortunate passing led to the real beginning of my pharmacy career. I was chosen to assist as a clerk in the pharmacy section of the store. Remember, this was before self-service. When you went shopping at the drugstore, you told the clerk what items you wished to purchase, and the clerk went to each section of the store to retrieve your purchases . . . then bring the items back to the service counter, ring the sale on the cash register, and then wrap the items and tie them with string. This was before cellophane tape was invented, and paper sacks were not commonly used.

While clerking behind the pharmacy service counter, I can remember just as if it were yesterday, I sold my first bottle of REM cough syrup along with a box of Bromo- Quinine cold tablets to a person with a cough and cold. Other cold and cough products of the day were 4 Way Cold Tablets, Pertussin Cough Syrup, Cherry Bark or Creosote based cough syrups. Also, there were bottles of the popular VonDrasek's Laxative Cold Capsules.

All the above-mentioned cough and cold products were later proved not too effective in treating colds and coughs, but they were the regime of the day. So, this is what people used at the time.

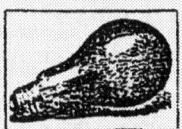

SIDE LITES

For as long as I can remember, it's been said that if you treat a cold it will last seven days . . . if you don't, the cold will go away in one week..

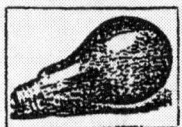

Friend: John has the Egyptian flu.
Joe: I've never heard of the Egyptian flu. Where did he get it?
Friend: He got it from his Mummy.

Late one winter evening a customer came back to the pharmacy service counter to purchase a cough and cold product, and during the sale he said to me, "Son, what the world really needs is a better mousetrap and a cure for the common cold." As we all know better mousetraps are continuously being developed, but the ever-elusive cure for the common cold has yet to be found. Upon hearing that cough and cold customer's statement for the first time, I was struck with an obsession, not to create a better mousetrap, but to find a cure for the common cold.

In 1946 I applied for and received my State of Illinois Pharmacy Apprentice license, and in 1949 I applied for and entered pharmacy school at the University of Illinois. I graduated in 1953. I was the first on either side of the family to attend college. Soon after graduation I entered the military service for two years with most of that time stationed at a major Army hospital. It was there I trained and practiced as a hospital laboratory technician. This gave me an excellent opportunity to further my knowledge of the medical field. Even with all my military duties, I found time to work as a part time pharmacist in a small local retail pharmacy in a near by town. During my pharmacy career, which spanned over 56 years, I worked at, managed, and/or supervised over 150 pharmacies and drugstores in Illinois, Washington, Alaska, Montana, Idaho, and Oregon.

During the last ten years of my pharmacy career I was the Director of Pharmacy Operations of a division of a national supermarket chain. At the time of retirement I was in charge of 131 pharmacy operations. This position was mainly an office job, and during those ten years the thing I missed most was the contact with prescription patients I had while managing or working in a pharmacy. Not only did I miss the contact with the prescription patients, but also the satisfaction of assisting them with their health and health needs. Over the years I was able to aid many customers and prescription patients in smoking cessation, lowering cholesterol and high blood pressure levels, and lose many pounds on sensible diets. *All this was done with recommendations that were natural and required no pills or medications.*

In March of 2000, I retired from the practice of pharmacy at near age 70.

THE OFFERING

GOOD NEWS - a Seattle pharmacist discovers an amazing and natural way to prevent the common cold and flu.

STOP HAVING ALL THOSE BOUTS WITH COLDS AND FLU.

Why suffer all those cold and flu miseries? Look, feel, and be healthier!

I can remember the miserable feeling of a stuffy nose and the horrible look of a runny nose . . . those cold chills and fever . . . congested ears . . . that scratchy sore throat . . . that all over aching feeling . . . the difficult breathing. Oh, how terrible I felt when catching a cold or experiencing a bout with the flu. And what about the other illnesses that can follow, often referred to as secondary infections or complications: ear and sinus infections, pneumonia, bronchitis, and asthma attacks. Colds and flu can be very devastating to you, a family member, a friend, or anyone.

MAKE THE COMMON COLD AND FLU UNCOMMON TO YOU.

I no longer catch those 2 or 3 colds a year like I used to. Also, I no longer get bouts of the flu. Now it's great to be one of the 4 to 6% of Americans who seldom catch a cold or the flu. While following my own anti-cold and flu method, I haven't had a bout with the flu since 1970. The people I have revealed my anti-viral method to have experienced the same unbelievable results. Now you, your family, and your friends, like all those who have learned of and followed my anti-viral method, can also become one of the coveted 4-6%. All you have to do is follow the health advice I'm willing to share with you. The anti-viral method is so natural and easy to follow anyone can do it! I discovered this anti-viral method by accident after years of research and experimentation. It's so simple and uncomplicated, I just can't figure out why some research scientist or other person in the health profession has not uncovered it before.

IT'S UNBELIEVABLE!   IT'S EASY!   IT'S NATURAL!

No prescription drugs or medicines are required. Just what is required? The special know how that was discovered, and I am willing to share with you. My anti-viral method is a must for anyone who wants to lead a healthier more productive life . . . you, your family, your friends, athletes, business people, teachers, health professionals, senior citizens, and etc., etc., etc.

To obtain your copy of *The J. Albert Anti-Viral Report* simply fill out and send me the special money saving introductory order blank below along with $20 plus $5 for shipping and handling. You'll save $10 off the $30 cover price. You'll have to agree that $20 is a small price to pay to make the common cold and flu uncommon to you and with all those with whom you share this information. Prevent just one bout with a cold or flu for your family and you'll save more than your investment in *The J. Albert Anti-Viral Report*. And think of all the misery and suffering you can prevent. This health report is a must for bronchitis and asthma sufferers who may suffer severe attacks brought on by colds and flu. THERE WILL PROBABLY NEVER BE A CURE FOR THE COMMON COLD OR FLU, BUT WHAT DIFFERENCE WHEN BOTH CAN BE PREVENTED!

For those who might be skeptical of this offer, here are a few of the many unsolicited testimonials pertaining to my advice and health methods.

I'M HEALTHIER NOW!

After following J. Albert's advice I haven't had a cold or bout with the flu for 4 1/2 years. Till that time I had one cold or bout with the flu after another. I even ended up in the hospital several times in a one year time frame. J. Albert's advice is the greatest!

—Mr. M.W., Puyallup, WA

ASK YOUR PHARMACIST.

J. Albert's advice on colds and flu is priceless. I've had excellent advice from a top-notch pharmacist.

—Mr. A.G., Tacoma, WA

TAKE STOCK IN YOUR HEALTH

When J. Albert speaks about health, people should listen.

—Mrs. M.T., Renton, WA

THANK YOU J. ALBERT.

Since J. Albert shared his anti-viral method with me, my wife and I haven't had a cold or flu for 4 years. While spending last winter in Phoenix, my wife and I were the only retirees of our group of friends that didn't have the flu during a season of epidemic proportions.

—Mr. S.D., Seattle, WA

BE HEALTHIER AND SAVE MONEY.

Following J. Albert's advice on colds and flu has resulted in a healthier life for my family. It also lowered my medical and prescription bills.

—Mr. D.J., Tacoma, WA

LIFE-SAVING ADVICE!

J. Albert's information on colds and flu most likely saved my life.

—Mr. R.M., Seattle, WA

YOU CAN COUNT ON J. ALBERT.

J. Albert is always ready to take time to share his wealth of health advice.

—Mrs. E.J., Seattle, WA

(Initials are used for sake of privacy . . . Names are on file)

ACT NOW to obtain your copy of "The J. Albert Anti-Viral Report." You'll have to agree that $20 plus $5 for shipping and handling is a small price to pay to make the common cold and flu uncommon to you and those with whom you'll share this information.

THE ABOVE ADVERTISING MESSAGE WAS FOLLOWED RIGHT HERE WITH AN ORDER BLANK TO ORDER YOUR COPY OF THE "THE J. ALBERT ANTIVIRAL REPORT."

What you have just read was an advertisement I first wrote in 1983, so I could share my anti-viral discovery with others, and what you have just read is what this book is about and the information that will be shared with you. However, because of astronomical startup and advertising costs, the project was abandoned.

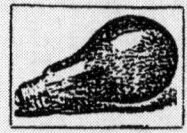

SIDE LITE

You may ask why I would charge a price for such valuable health information. Well, I found over my years of serving the public, and it seems to be human nature, that if you don't charge for information you give or include the information with the sale of a product, people perceive it to be of no value and won't follow it. Put a price on it, or sell it as part of a package—WHAMO! Those who pay for the info will most likely follow the advice given.

The anti-viral information was shared with a couple of pharmaceutical companies and an assistant dean at one of the local professional colleges. Little interest was shown, so I packed up my information and stored it away.

I would like you to know that I didn't hide this anti-viral information from anyone. It was continually shared with my pharmacy patients and customers along with friends, relatives, and fellow employees.

Another interesting fact that I have found in human nature is that "family most often will not listen to family." With the information you'll receive in this book, you'll probably have to do a "hard sell" to get other family members to follow it. Better yet, let them read this book on their own and come to their own conclusions.

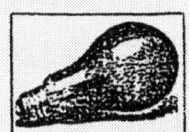

SIDE LITE

FAMILY PERSUASION During a pharmacy convention I attended a few years back, a dermatologist told a story about his teenage daughter. It seems her skin was "breaking out" with facial blemishes. On seeing this, he advised her how to address the situation to clear her complexion. She didn't follow his advice. Her facial blemishes continued. Then about 6 months later her skin almost miraculously cleared. She now had that glowing "peaches and cream complexion." He was amazed! He asked his daughter what she did to clear up her face. She told him she had read a health article on problem skin in one of the monthly women's magazines. She followed the recommended procedure on how to have healthy looking, blemish free skin. He was very happy for her. *LITTLE DID SHE KNOW THAT THE ARTICLE ON A BETTER LOOKING COMPLEXION WAS WRITTEN BY THE DOCTOR HIMSELF.* He did mention that he never told his daughter that he wrote the article for the magazine.

NOW READ ON TO LEARN MORE ABOUT "THE OFFERING" ON ALL I HAVE PRESENTED TO YOU IN THIS CHAPTER.

The J. Albert
Anti-Viral Report
(Updated 2006)

"Research is to see what everybody else has seen, and to think what nobody else has thought."

—ALBERT SZENT-GYÖRGY

The J. Albert Anti-Viral Report

WHAT I AM about to reveal to you I first became aware of over 20 years ago. Actually, the events which led to this began almost 6 years prior. Let me start there.

It was a hot summer day in July in Seattle. There was not a cloud in the sky. The sun was hot and the temperature was 92° F on the tennis court.

SIDE LITES

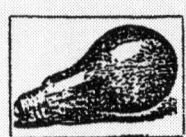 It's true that Seattle receives more than its share of rain; however, its summer days can be beautiful. It's been said that people in Seattle don't tan . . . they rust.

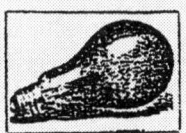 And it was Mark Twain who said the finest winter he ever spent was a summer on the Puget Sound.

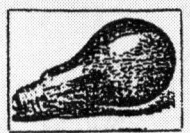 And how is a 40% chance of rain predicted by your weatherperson? I've been told the answer to that it's when 4 out 10 weatherpersons say it's going to rain.

I was sweating profusely, and as the tennis match proceeded my legs began to "ache." I played through the discomfort and as usual lost the matches to my next- door neighbor, a high school athletic coach. After the matches while walking back to our homes, I mentioned to him that during the tennis match I developed "aching legs." His comment to this was that possibly the lack of potassium in my system could be the underlying cause of the aches I experienced.

The very same day I drove over to the local supermarket to purchase a bottle of juice that was high in potassium content. I began to drink a three ounce glass twice daily. The results . . . over a short period of time my leg muscle soreness went away.

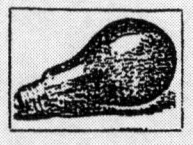

SIDE LITE

QUESTION? Don't you think as a pharmacist I should have known that I was lacking potassium in my system? I did, but I'll have to admit at the time I didn't think of it.

Because I enjoyed the juice, it became a regular daily part of my diet. It was a little later when I noticed that I was not catching my usual bouts of cold or flu. I attributed this to the daily vitamin I was taking at this time. After all, as a pharmacist, colds and flu were considered an occupational hazard due to the fact that there was continual contact with people seeking advice on colds and flu or filling their prescriptions for such. Over a 32-year time frame I've had four or five colds. And to the best of my recollection, I believe the illnesses happened at a time when the juice was not part of my regular diet. Also, there is another reason for me "catching a cold", which I will further address later in this report.

There were times, in the drugstores and pharmacies I practiced in, that every pharmacy employee but myself came down with flu. Some were so ill they missed several days of work. This was a time when there was no such thing as paid sick leave, and many of these pharmacy employees could not afford to miss work.

The juice I was DRINKING and still drink daily today is grape juice. That's grape juice, not grapefruit juice. You know, grape juice . . . the purple stuff.

In March of 1977 a news article appeared at about the same time in the *Tacoma News Tribune* and *The Seattle Times* newspapers that played up the fact that wine and grape juice contain ingredients that inhibit viruses.

Read them for yourself.

To your health!

A little vino good for viruses, studies show.

ABOVE WAS A title of a news article written by Joel N. Shurkin for the Knight News Service and appeared in the *Seattle Times* newspaper in March of 1977.

Due to not being able to receive permission to reprint the article; I'll highlight the presentation with bullet points.

- the article went on to state that two Canadian scientists discovered that red wine can kill several viruses that can cause disease.

- the research work was performed for the Canadian Health and Welfare Agency's Bureau of Microbial Hazards.

- it was found that wine, strawberries, and raspberries contain antiviral properties.

- discovered was wine and various fruit extracts killed the polio virus, the cold sore causing virus, a type of meningitis, and upset stomach causing viruses.

- the antiviral properties were traced to chemicals called phenols, especially found in grape skin.

- red wine contains more phenols than white wine, however, red grape juice is the strongest in antiviral phenol containing properties.

The news article also mentioned that ancient soldiers mixed wine with water to purify it to prevent the Mediterranean version of "La Tourista."

Attack of the grape leaves viruses weak

WASHINGTON (AP) — *The medicinal value of grapes and wine, long touted in folklore of many countries, is getting a boost from science with the discovery that grapes kill viruses.*

For centuries, people worldwide have praised the healing benefits of the grape. Roman soldiers use to pour wine into wounds and ancient Egyptian warriors mixed wine with the unfamiliar water of countries they invaded.

Although known for many years that wine kills bacteria, Canadian scientists only recently discovered the antiviral properties.

In a report to the journal Applied and Environmental Microbiology, researchers for the Canadian Department of Health and Welfare in Ottawa say grapes, grape juice, raisins and wines show antiviral activity in the test tube.

Microbiologists Dr. Jack Konowalchuk and Joan I. Speirs said grapes and grape juice were stronger viral killers than wines. And in every case, red wines were more potent against viruses than white wines.

The researchers said there was not a way of knowing how these test-tube results might apply to human health. But all the viruses in the experiments were those that affect humans, such as herpes simplex and poliovirus, which cause herpes infections and polio.

"It is not the policy of the government to advocate drinking wine or anything else," Konowalchuk said in an interview Thursday. "But judging from these results, I would say grape juice is a very beneficial drink."

The researchers said the antibacterial properties of wine have been attributed to natural chemicals found in grapes, such as tannic acid and phenols.

Konowalchuk said he suspects the phenols may affect the viruses by binding to them and preventing them from infecting cells and multiplying.

—The News Tribune, Tacoma
    March 4, 1977

(Reprinted by permission of the Associated Press)

Even before reading the info in the two articles above, one must remember that nature provides many medicinal properties from which drugs have been derived to assist mankind to live a healthier productive life. As examples there's quinine, which is extracted from the bark of the cinchona tree which is used to treat malaria. For heart ailments there's digitalis derived from the foxglove plants. And let's not forget penicillin, which is a product of common mold, or opium which is obtained from the poppy plant. Also, there's an anticancer drug prepared from an extract from the Pacific Yew tree bark. The list goes on and on. Even today new discoveries for the use of natural products are being uncovered.

I've had prescription patients who years ago lowered their cholesterol levels by 15 to 20 per cent by just eating oatmeal daily at breakfast. And just recently researchers at the Beltsville Human Nutrition Center in Maryland ran a study and found that by supplementing a quarter teaspoonful of cinnamon into the diets of people with diabetes, they lowered glucose, fat, and cholesterol levels by as much as 30%.

As part of a $2.5 million five-year university grant, researchers are currently studying folklore cures of people in Latin America, Southeast Asia, and Africa. Another university band of researchers is off to the Highland Maya people of Mexico where many vascular plant species can be found. These research scientists are sure their findings will unveil new plant wonder drugs. I learned of this from an article in the winter issue 1999/2000 of *Back to Health* magazine.

Outside of natural immunity and/or not being exposed to the cold or flu virus, the most likely reason SOME don't catch the common cold or flu during outbreaks of the disease is one, they probably practice excellent personal hygiene and two, and most likely, they either knowingly or unknowingly as part of their diets consume Mother Nature's own anti-viral preventatives in such products as grape juice, wine, or other STILL UN-KNOWN anti-viral containing food products.

It goes without saying that I have continued to drink and advocate the daily drinking of grape juice. Those who have followed my daily recommendation and also take a daily multivitamin have unbelievable results.

Yes, that's right. I did mention the recommendation of a daily multivitamin to go along with the grape juice. For about twenty years the medical practice didn't recommend vitamins as a dietary supplement. It was professed that all one had to do is eat a balanced diet to obtain all the vitamins one needed. It was contended that all vitamin taking did was create very expensive urine.

With this sort of statement by the medical profession it made it a challenge for me to get many of my pharmacy patients and others to take a daily multivitamin. However, in June of 2002, the American Medical Association did an about face and published an article declaring most Americans should take a daily multivitamin for their specific age group for chronic disease prevention. There are multivitamins for infants, children, adults, seniors, etc. To meet your specific needs, ask your physician or pharmacist for a multivitamin recommendation.

How long have I taken daily multivitamins? For about 58 years. That's since I was about 17 years old.

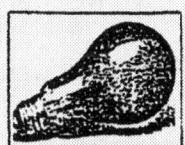

SIDE LITES

I've mentioned how important I feel vitamins are for one's health, and people often ask me what vitamin products I take myself. Although my vitamin preferences have changed from time to time over the years due to various changes in formulation by the drug companies, I presently take one multivitamin daily that is for a person 50 years or older. *That's right; all I take for vitamins is one multivitamin tablet daily.* There are many people who take many vitamins daily. In my opinion unless otherwise professionally advised, they are wasting their money. Not sure what vitamin products to take...again, check with your pharmacist or doctor for a suggestion. People with special needs or medical conditions are recommended to check with their doctor.

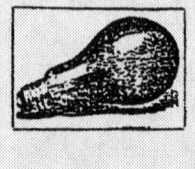 I want you to know that in my long pharmacy career, I would never, that's right never, recommend any health product that I wouldn't use or recommend for my family or myself. There were many times when people would bring a product to purchase to the prescription counter. I would tell them not to use that product, and put it back. Only if they insisted, would I then sell them the item or product.

SO NOW IT'S GRAPE JUICE AND A DAILY MULTIVITAMIN TO PROTECT ONE FROM GETTING A COLD OR FLU.

Let me give you just four of many case histories of those whom I have given the J. Albert anti-cold and flu advice.

CASE #1 . . . Bill M.

Bill M. is a white male in his middle seventies. Bill is a music instrument repairman in a music store in the same shopping center where I managed a pharmacy. He constantly had bouts with colds and flu, which more often than not led to secondary pulmonary infections. He would suffer such a bout on the average of every eight to ten weeks. With each illness Bill would consume a ten day supply of the current popular antibiotic plus several bottles of an antihistaminic codeine expectorant cough syrup. In one year, he had to be admitted to the local hospital several times for a few days.

I was concerned about Bill's health, so one day I took Bill off to the side and away from the prescription counter. I asked him whether he would consider following some free health advice on colds and flu. His answer was affirmative. He said he would follow any advice to stop all the battles with colds and flu.

I proceeded to tell him of the daily multivitamin and glass of grape juice I consumed each day. Bill said he was already taking the same multivitamin tablet I was, and he agreed to make grape juice part of his daily diet.

What were Bill's results? For 4 1/2 years he didn't have a cold or flu. I transferred to another pharmacy location for the company I was employed and didn't see Bill again for about another 4 years at which time he excitedly came up to me and said he was still having the same results . . . NO COLDS . . . NO FLU . . . NO HOSPITAL STAYS. Bill was 85 at our last meeting and was still holding down a full time job.

CASE #2 . . . Leona C.

Leona C. is a white middle-aged woman who was very susceptible to asthmatic and bronchitis attacks, which were most often brought on by the common cold. In fact, just about any "bug" that came around would infect her. Leona would require an expensive batch of antibiotic prescriptions every six to eight weeks.

After making her aware of my grape juice and multivitamin regime, Leona took my advice to heart and followed the advice I gave her. She couldn't believe the results. For ten months she didn't have one cold or bout with the flu. After this ten-month time frame, she moved out of the area, and I lost contact with her.

GRAPE JUICE AND A DAILY MULTIVITAMIN ARE A MUST FOR ALL WHO SUFFER ASTHMA AND BRONCHITIS ATTACKS.

CASE #3 . . . Mr. C.J.

C.J. is a white male and was about 65 years old when I first met him. He was a very high profile division manager of a huge food and drug combination supermarket chain. I first met C.J. when he transferred into the same division of the company where I was employed as the Director of Pharmacy Operations.

However, before I met C.J., my counterpart in the division of the company C.J. transferred from informed me to keep an ample supply of cough and cold products in my office for C.J. The informant told me that every time C.J. came down with a cold or flu, the first place he would head for was the pharmacy director for advice plus a "handful of suitable pills and a bottle of cough syrup."

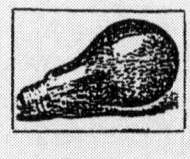

SIDE LITE

It was quite common for most anyone in the division to visit my office for my advice and opinion on matters of health. Why not? My advice was free. After getting my advice or opinion, I would jokingly tell them as they were leaving there was no charge for the office call.

The first week C.J. arrived in the division, I had the opportunity to tell him my anti-viral approach to colds and flu. It interested him immensely. In his opinion it sounded like an easy, simple, and natural way to prevent colds and flu.

He began to follow the advice. Only once over a five year period did he visit my office for some advice and some medication for a cold. He came down with a severe cold in the middle of a mild cold and flu season. During our conversation he admitted he wasn't drinking his daily glass of grape juice before bedtime for a few weeks. C.J. received a promotion to the corporate office. Seeing him on one of his later visits to the division, he told me he still follows my anti-cold and flu advice with all the same great results . . . NO COLDS . . . AND NO BOUTS WITH THE FLU. C.J.'s wife, on our last meeting, referred to me as his "doctor."

You may be wondering where all the cold and flu medications came from that I had in my office. Actually, they were samples of the latest or newest over-the-counter products that salespersons would give me to introduce new cold and flu products. Cold and cough products are one of the largest selling categories in the drug department today.

Case #4...J. ALBERT

That's right. Though out this book I have or will reveal to you my own successes while following my own advice.

MANY, MANY OTHERS WHO HAVE HEARD THE SAME RECOMMENDATION AND FOLLOWED IT HAVE HAD THE SAME BENEFICIAL HEALTH RESULTS AS BILL M., LEONA C., MR. C.J., AND ME.

In 1952, when I was a senior in pharmacy school at the University of Illinois, our class took a physiology class with freshman medical students. During the year, a lecture was given on colds and flu and the effects they had on people. The lecturer revealed to the class one of his personal observations . . . an observation, which completely baffled him. As a doctor in the Emergency Room of Cook County Hospital, he treated many of the street people or homeless for various mishaps and illnesses.

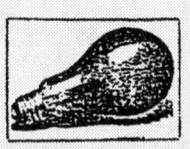

SIDE LITE

At the time I attended pharmacy school, Cook County Hospital was just kitty-corner from the University of Illinois Medical, Dental, and Pharmacy Schools near downtown Chicago. The newly located hospital is the fictional setting for the T.V. series *E.R.*

In the 1950's the people we now call "street people" or "the homeless" were called "bums" and "hobos" and resided in the doorways and in and on the curbs of West Madison Street which was very near the hospital. The thing that for him was something of a wonderment was that no matter what time of year or weather conditions prevailed outside, he saw very few of these people with colds or flu. He just couldn't figure it out. Remember, Chicago can be very hot in the summer and very, very cold in the winter. Having spent two years in Fairbanks, Alaska, I can attest to the fact that I felt colder in Chicago at 6° F above zero than in Fairbanks at 59° F below zero.

Looking back on the good doctor's amazement, it's now easy to see why these people seldom caught a cold or flu. *They received their "grape juice" in the form of wine...muscatel, port, sherry, or any other kind of wine available to them.* These people were also called "winos" in those days.

Now, just how does drinking grape juice prevent colds and flu? To answer this question I must refer to my unbelievable encounter with the *"green covered book."*

During one of my many visits to the local library to continue my never-ending search for colds and flu information, I came upon a copy of a *"green covered book"* whose title I can't remember. This was 1983 and years before the Internet. The book with a green cover was about the common cold with the author revealing his experiences with such.

Most often on visits to his parents on a Sunday evening his two children came down with a cold just a few days later. Most often on departing from the grandparents' on those visit each child was given a piece of candy. The author of the book with the green cover surmised that the candy set up a condition in the throats of the children to allow the infection of a cold virus.

Now you may ask, where's the mystery? Well, after scanning the *green covered book* only one time that night, it could never be located again at the library. I went back several times over a six-month time frame to find this publication. I combed the stacks, searched the card file for clues with assistance from several different librarians. The searches were futile and all to no avail.

It was like the book with the green cover was placed in the local library one night, one and only one night, for my review and revelation. What revelation and answer did I find? The answer was how grape juice prevents colds and flu in people. I had my one and only chance, and luck was with me. The two newspaper articles that you have read previously along with the Sunday night story of the two children unfolded the solution to me—***how and where grape juice works to inhibit viral growth.***

The throat and nasal passages are where the virus invades and incubates in people. After being infected by the virus it takes about 2-1/2 to 3 days for the cold & flu symptoms to appear. Just how does grape juice prevent colds and flu? It most likely binds with or inactivates the virus and in some manner prevents it from spreading throughout one's system. It's so simple! As you have read in the two news articles previously presented grape juice contains nature's own antiviral properties. And again, as one drinks the juice the antiviral properties contained within may bind with the cold and flu virus to inactivate them. Further research will be required to exactly prove how grape juice actually accomplishes its antiviral action.

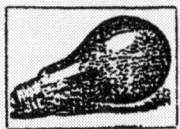

SIDE LITE

In the late 50's and early 60's drug companies promoted treatments for colds that contained natural bioflavonoid. I sold hundreds of packages of these products. However, the products proved ineffective. The bioflavonoid contained in the cold product is similar to the ingredients in grape juice. They are antiviral. Why do the antiviral properties of grape juice prevent colds and flu while the marketed products of the 50's and 60's did not? First of all, the medication was in capsule form and passed the throat where the infection starts. And second and most important the product was used after the cold symptoms appeared and had already spread throughout the body.

IMPORTANT REMINDER

As stated in the Preface, when a vitamin or vitamins are mentioned throughout this book, I am referring to a combination of both vitamins and minerals...a MULTIVITAMIN/MULTIMINERAL SUPPLEMENT. Balances of minerals, like vitamins, are essential for insurance of a healthy diet.
With any special health need or needs, it's recommended you check with your health provider for the proper product or products to use.

NATURE HAS A SOLUTION FOR EVERY SITUATION.... ALL ONE HAS TO DO IS DISCOVER IT.

—J. Albert

As mentioned earlier this also explains why some people in a group catch colds and flu when others do not. Outside of practicing other hygienic preventions such as frequent hand washing and avoiding crowds during out breaks of colds and flu, those who did not become infected with the virus even though exposed, most likely drank or ate some food or beverage that inactivated the virus and prevented infection.

One must remember this antiviral method prevents colds and flu. It does not cure them. Once the infection takes hold and spreads throughout one's body, IT'S TOO LATE!! I can't count the number of times people have mentioned to me that after they came down with the flu or a cold, they started drinking grape juice.

Again, the J. Albert anti-viral method only prevents the common cold and flu. It does not cure either. This is the reason why IT IS VITAL TO drink your grape juice daily. It's A PRE-VENTATIVE MEASURE.

Many have asked why take a daily multivitamin? My answer has and always will be, it's insurance. It's insurance that you receive the nutrients you need to maintain a healthy diet. That's right . . . it's insurance.

I have already revealed to you the method by which you, your family, your friends and all those you tell can live a life with fewer colds and bouts with the flu. Let's face it! Occasionally there's a breakdown and one of the two bugs may strike. However, such incidents will be few and far between. TO PREVENT GETTING A BOUT WITH A COLD OR FLU, IT'S AS EASY AS 1, 2, and there is no 3.

Here again for a matter of review and simplification is:

THE J. ALBERT ANTI-COLD & FLU METHOD

1. Each day take a multivitamin product suitable for your age group. Although it's not needed for the antiviral protection, the vitamin is extra insurance.

2. Everyday before bedtime and ten minutes before you brush your teeth drink grape juice.

3. LIKE I SAID, THERE IS NO #3. THAT'S ALL THERE IS TO IT!

Just how much grape juice is enough to drink each night at bedtime?

•   For those ages 12 and older drink a minimum of 3 ounces daily.

•   For those ages 6 through 11 drink a minimum of 2 ounces daily.

- For those ages 3 through 5 drink 1 ounce daily.

FOR CHILDREN UNDER 3 YEARS OF AGE, CHECK WITH YOUR DOCTOR OR PEDIATRICIAN FOR QUANTITIES OF GRAPE JUICE TO DRINK.

Doesn't it seem so easy? For the life of me I just can't figure out why no one has discovered this before. In this case it can be said that people probably just couldn't "see the trees for the forest" or was it "the forest for the trees" whichever way the saying goes. I could never remember which way was which.

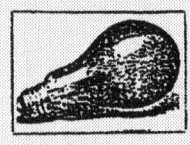

SIDE LITE

Another benefit of drinking grape juice daily that I have found was not having stomach aches or upsets. I never had too many, but while drinking grape juice daily I haven't had any at all. The occasional mouth sores I use to get are also now nonexistent. And as for cold sores on my lips, at the first sign of that tingling sensation caused by the virus, I would rub my tongue over the tingling area after drinking my nightly grape juice. By morning the tingling sensation is gone and no cold sores appear.

Just because you now have a method to prevent the common cold and flu, there is no reason not to continue the everyday practices to prevent getting or transmitting both. In life to stay healthy you have to "stack the deck" any way you can. It's just plain common sense.

Here are just a few of the many ways to prevent getting or spreading the cold and flu viruses. A few of the ways will just be reminders. Some will be new. Here they are.

1. Wash your hands frequently, and that's with soap and water. If no soap or water are available, use one of the hand sanitizers now commercially available.

SIDE LITES

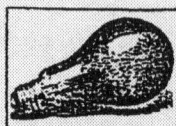

In one branch of the military service all the recruits were ordered to wash their hands at least five times a day. The result was 40-50% fewer bouts of respiratory sickness among this group of troops versus others. Hand washing has been recommended as an easy way to stop the spread of infectious disease for over 100 years.

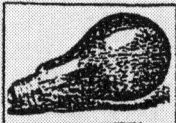

As an introductory statement to a microbiology class I took in pharmacy school, the instructor stated that after the class concluded, not only will you wash your hands after you go the bath room, you'll also wash your hands before you go.

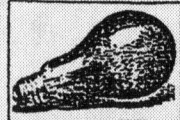

Very recently I saw a little sign above the wash basin in the men's room of a fast food restaurant reminding all to wash their hands rubbing the hands together with soap and water for at least ten seconds before rinsing. Just how long is ten seconds? Sing one verse of *Happy Birthday* to yourself. That's ten seconds!

I often wonder how much less illness there would be if all restroom doors opened out instead of having to be pulled to leave. Think of all the times you wouldn't have to pull a handle of the restroom door . . . a handle that is pulled many times a day by people who, after relieving themselves, do not wash their hands. Many places now have a press plate you can brush up against to open the restroom door. Some hospitals recommend that their employees, after washing their hands and drying them with paper towels, use the paper towels to open the restroom doors. Now many of the nation's airports, malls, and sporting facilities have the right idea . . . many restrooms with no doors at all.

Before eating, handling, or preparing food be sure to wash your hands for 20 seconds. That's right...sing two versus of *Happy Birthday*.

NOW ALL THIS ISN'T JUST ABOUT WASHING YOUR HANDS AFTER USING THE BATHROOM FACILITIES, IT'S ABOUT WASHING YOUR HANDS THROUGH OUT THE DAY. THIS IS ESPECIALLY ESSENTIAL DURING THE COLD AND FLU SEASON, BECAUSE THESE VIRAL INFECTIONS ARE SPREAD BY CONTACT WITH ANOTHER PERSON OR BY PERSON TO OBJECT TO PERSON CONTACT.

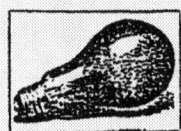

SIDE LITE

Over many years of prescription filling I noticed a pattern that occurred in the late winter and early spring. Approximately three days after the first nice days of weather where children would be able to play outside and adults would take advantage to start their early gardening for the year, the cold virus would run rampant and infect many. How did I know this? Well, people would flock to the pharmacy to have their prescriptions filled for colds and flu symptoms. Remember, this was at a time when doctors prescribed antibiotics for just about any type of infection including colds and flu. **As most know now, antibiotics are not effective for viral infections, and over the past decade the number of prescriptions written for antibiotics to treat colds is becoming less and less**.

Then it dawned on me! Many viruses and bacteria "brew" in the soil over the winter months. The children who played outside, the early gardener and many who took advantage of the good early weather exposed themselves to the viruses. Not only might they become infected, but also they may spread the infection to others. It was a bonanza for the pharmacy business.

With the weather conditions turning dismal again for a time and another nice day or days return, the same would happen again. Not till early May when the sun had time to kill the viruses and bacteria in the soil did the infections subside. For the early gardener I always recommended wearing gloves while working the soil and for children and others outside on these early great days of weather, be sure to wash hands frequently.

These findings were for the Seattle area and most likely will differ from area to area depending on local weather.

> Another thing I observed over the years was that after extreme prolonged periods of dry weather, colds, flu, and other illnesses become more prevalent and severe when the windy wet weather returns. I've often wondered if the earth's water table had something to do with this. It's a thought.

2. Keep your hands away from your face. A virus can infect a person when touching a contaminated hand or finger to the eyes, nose or mouth. Most viruses that cause colds and flu are spread by direct contact. For example, when you sneeze into your hand an then touch an object such as a telephone, drinking glass, a computer keyboard, etc. the germs can live for hours or up to a week and can infect the next person who touches the viral or bacterial contaminated item.

3. During times of cold and flu outbreaks avoid crowds whenever possible.

4. Get enough sleep and rest. Eight hours of sleep each night is recommended.

5. Be sure to eat a balanced diet that includes lots of fruits and vegetables. Don't forget your daily vitamin.

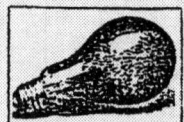

SIDE LITE

Years ago I worked with a pharmacist who was a chronic "junk food" eater. He very seldom sat down and ate a regular meal. It was just snack, snack, and snack some more. I often reminded him "you are what you eat." His retort to me was always "What did you have to eat on THANKSGIVING DAY?"

6. Do all that is possible to reduce your stress levels. Stress can weaken the immune system. Yoga, meditation, and exercise can be great stress reducers.

SIDE LITES

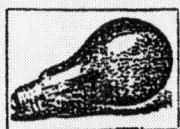

Many years ago I read a magazine article, which addressed the life span of the worker bee in a bee-hive. After many years of research it was found that worker bees that produced work in the hive lived longer than ones who did little or no work. Is there a corollary between bees and humans? I believe so for I read again and again in health articles that people who perform physical work or the equivalent with forms of exercise, not only have a better quality of life now and in their later years, but also have a greater life expectancy. I can remember my father-in-law saying, "SON, AS LONG AS YOU KEEP MOVING THEY CAN'T BURY YOU." I guess there is truth to what he used to say.

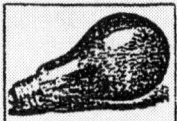

I want you to know that fitness didn't become part of my personal health program till I was about 46 years old. It was at that time I started a jogging and workout program. About 14 years later while talking with one of my prescription patients about his health, I recommended he start an exercise program. I told him by doing so now at age 60 I'm in better physical shape than when I was 30. He looked me over a few seconds and retorted, "Gee, you must have been in terrible physical shape when you were 30."

7.   Don't share drinking or eating utensils with family members or others who may have a cold or flu.

8.   Before brushing your teeth always rinse your toothbrush under the faucet with running water. That includes the whole brush . . . the bristles and handle. This can rinse off any contamination on the brush.

9.   As mentioned in the following SIDE LITE, if your home heating and cooling system utilizes a replaceable furnace filter that is sold at most discount and hardware stores,

I highly endorse their use. The filters can reduce harmful airborne particles including mold, bacteria, pollen, and dust *particles, which can carry the cold and flu viruses.*

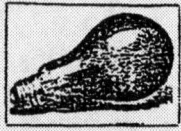

SIDE LITE

There are many types of replaceable furnace filters in the market. They range from the very inexpensive in cost, which in my opinion are almost the same as using no filter at all, to the top of the line filters, which I highly recommend. For years I used in our home an inexpensive filter. Then on the recommendation of a pharmacist I was working with I installed one of the best filters on the market. The first noticeable thing was the absence of dust throughout our home. Our home became practically "dust free." The inexpensive filters filter the air mechanically as it passes through the filter. The top of the line filters trap particles both mechanically and electrostatically making the filter much more efficient by filtering smaller particle contaminants from the air. If you can't use a disposable furnace filter in your home, I highly suggest using one of the many room air filters and purifier machines in the market. Check them out. It's important to have clean air in your home.

10.   DON"T SMOKE!!! This is for all the obvious reasons, and the fact that smoking can lower your resistants to colds and flu.

And last but not least.

11.   For #11 I am reminding you again of #1. Remember to wash your hands frequently!!! . . . Frequently wash your hands!!! . . . Wash your hands frequently at least six times a day!!! More is even better! *Recently I read a newspaper article that stated the reason SARS, Severe Acute Respiratory Syndrome, didn't spread throughout Taiwan and Japan like other countries was that the people of these nations frequently wash their hands.*

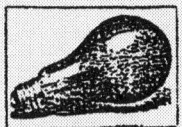

SIDE LITE

Let's face it. Luck plays a part in life. Being at the wrong place at the wrong time can expose a person to the cold and flu virus. However, following a prevention program can reduce one's chance of infection.

When I reflect on luck I always think of my wife who is not a "gambler." She doesn't believe in luck and would never gamble or buy a lottery ticket. If I were to buy two lottery tickets and one ticket won 50 million dollars, she would most likely say to me why did you buy the other one. Anyway, don't gamble with your health! Do everything you can to maintain a healthy lifestyle.

I want you to know there was a time I had troubling doubts about the antiviral concept that I have just revealed to you . . . doubts that as a pharmacist I should have never had. However, somehow there must have been a reason for this dramatic turn of events. What reason I'll never know, however, these doubts and concerns led me to another major discovery to prevent illness. It was like somebody somehow, somewhere was sending me a message to pass on to all. Let me tell you about it.

The doubts of my antiviral program commenced early one year about the first week of April. One night I came home from a day's work in the pharmacy and began to feel ill with a scratchy sore throat. By bedtime that night I had a full- blown sore throat and my sinuses began to plug. By morning a fever added to my miseries. I thought to myself how could this happen? I've been drinking my grape juice each night. I've been taking my vitamins each morning. As the next day or so progressed, I ended up with a very nasty sinus infection, along with the sore throat and plugged ears. I felt terrible, so it was off to the doctor's office for a batch of prescriptions to fight the infection. What I had was a "head cold." Did you read what I just said . . . a "head cold?" Now hold that thought.

What I just described above happened about the time the major grape juice manufacturers discontinued bottling 100% Concord grape juice. The juice that was marketed had changed and was now produced from a concentrate.

Early in the fall of the same year the same episode repeated again. Another devastating "head cold" hit me. Only this time the throat and sinuses were very painful.

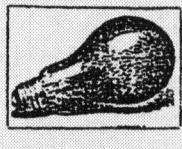

SIDE LITE

When pain is mentioned, I'm often reminded of the following story. At the age of ten one of my daughters persuaded my wife and I to let her have her ears pierced. This was long before body piercing was even thought of or in vogue. So, later that week we went down to the local mall for the piercing ritual. During the piercing of the first ear she let out a big "OUCH" and informed all within hearing range she now knows why there were so many pirates with only one earring. Oh, by the way, she did have the other ear pierced.

I fought the bug for about two weeks without any success. Again, it was off to the doc for another batch of prescriptions for the cure of this "head cold."

The only thing that I could figure out was going wrong was that the grape juice I was now drinking was produced from a concentrate rather than the 100% pure Concord grape juice. That had to be it, I decided. With that, I was off to find a store that still sold the 100% juice not produced from the concentrate. I found a couple of locations, and to this day **I drink only the 100% Concord grape juice that's not prepared from the concentrate**.

Another half year passed, and it's April again. You guessed it! Here came another repeat of the following year, or so I thought. It was a Wednesday night just before dinner when I felt the beginning of another "head cold" starting with the same scratchy sore throat. I thought to myself, "Oh no, not again!" I just knew I would be ill the next morning, just like before . . . another sore throat followed by another terrible sinus infection and more aching plugged ears.

It just happened that night that my wife and daughters were off to a mother-daughter affair, so I was left alone at home to prepare my own dinner. The dinner consisted of what use to be one of my favorites . . . two hot dogs with a little mustard. This time I noticed a fresh white peeled onion in the refrigerator, so I chopped up a portion of it and added it raw to the hot dogs. The raw onion was added to the hot dogs to give them that "baseball park taste."

I retired early that night. The next morning on awakening, I was amazed. Amazed was an understatement! I was astonished! I wasn't sick! Nothing happened! The scratchy throat wasn't sore. There were no symptoms of a sinus infection or plugged aching ears either.

What happened? The only thing different I did the night before was have the fresh chopped white onion on my hot dogs. I figured it had to be the onion that took care of the problem.

So that evening, after another day's work in the pharmacy it was off to the library to do a little research on onions. It didn't take very long to find out that one of the constituents of onions is allicin. And allicin is bacteriostatic in nature meaning it can inhibit the growth or kill bacteria. Years later I found many references stating the same on the Internet. An article published in the *Well-being Newsletter* by Loma Linda University titled "Garlic and Onions…Help Ward off Illness" stated the same. Further, I found that if it was heated, allicin breaks down and loses its bacteriostatic properties. And the last and most important finding was that the allicin in the onion, upon being eaten, sterilizes the throat, sinus, and ear passages within eight minutes.

The above finding accounted for my not becoming ill. It was the allicin contained in the fresh chopped raw onion on my hot dog I ate the night before for dinner that did the job. I've used this revelation or finding several times over the next few years, and it has worked. However, I'll have to admit that several times the process didn't work. What I found was that I needed to eat the fresh chopped raw onion within the first four hours of the first signs of a scratchy sore throat appearing. **IT HAS TO BE A FRESH WHITE ONION, NOT A YELLOW ONE OR ONE OF THE SWEET VARIETY.** Once the infection spreads or "took hold" it was too late. I prefer my onion treatment on a hot dog or as an onion sandwich.

SIDE LITES

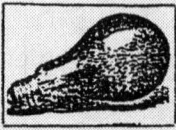

When thinking of time it reminds me of a shopping experience I had with my wife and father-in-law, a jeweler and watchmaker. While shopping for a picture to hang in our newly decorated recreation room, we came upon a beautiful painting of a Paris street scene. And on the corner of the street scene in the painting was a small clock on a pedestal. The clock in the picture actually kept time. The clock mechanism was behind the painting and was operated by a small battery. Both my wife and myself liked the painting very much, but we didn't purchase it. Why? It was because we took my father-in-law's advice. He said that if the clock ever broke or stopped running, we would have a picture that didn't work!

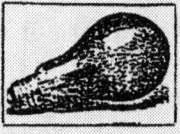

My father-in-law was only five foot four inches tall and always had humorous things to say. For example, he always said he didn't care how short he was just so his legs were long enough to reach the ground.

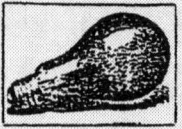

While on vacation and visiting the in-laws, my father-in-law had just come home for lunch from the jewelry store he owned and operated, at which time he announced to all at the dinner table that in the morning he sold a very young couple a "Canhardly Diamond" engagement ring. Not knowing, I asked him "What is a "Canhardly Diamond?" He explained to me that a "Canhardly Diamond" is a diamond so small you **can hardly** see it.

The information I've just shared with you has been shared with others over the years. They've had the same results I've had. They, like I, were amazed. You've probably noticed by now my use of the word amazed. Well, it's about the only way to describe my findings. It's so simple! It's so natural! It's so easy! It works! It's amazing!

Remember that thought I asked you to hold a few pages back about "head colds?" You most likely figured it out by now by yourself that a "head cold" is not a cold . . . it's an infection most often caused by a bacteria. Colds are viral in nature. That's why grape juice didn't prevent my sore throats, sinus, and/or ear infections. However, some of the above mentioned infections may be caused by a virus. So how do I know my infections were bacterial in nature? I deduced such, because I was drinking the antiviral grape juice.

Here I am, a pharmacist, and I should have known better; however, when I finally realized my misconception, it came to me that another method had been discovered that can prevent sore throats and sinus and ear infections . . . Mother Nature's own antibacterial principals in the raw white onion.

Another fantastic thing about this finding is that it can reduce the over usage of antibiotics greatly.

After the "onion find" I still continue to drink only the 100% Concord grape juice and not juice prepared from concentrate which most likely may still be effective in preventing colds and flu. However, I have no logical observations, research, or experimentation to conclude whether the juice prepared from the concentrate is or is not as effective. So why do I drink only the 100% Concord grape juice? It's because I enjoy the flavor and taste of the 100% Concord grape juice much more so than the juice prepared from concentrate.

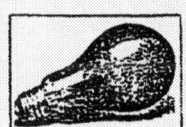

SIDE LITE

Another observation I made when I was infected with a sore throat and/or a sinus infection was that having an alcoholic drink made the infection worse. The same held true for cough or throat drops that contain menthol. This is just my own personal observation. The only conclusion that I can draw from this is that through time the bacteria causing the infections have adapted to the alcohol and menthol and are beginning to thrive on both. For this reason I recommend staying away from alcoholic beverages and menthol containing cough and cold products while suffering such infections.

Not long ago one of the major cough drop manufacturers introduced into the market a cough drop product eliminating menthol. And soon after another manufacturer did the same, and on its package in large letters proclaims "CONTAINS NO MENTHOL." I wonder why the change? What did these companies know? Or was this just another way to introduce an additional product to the public? Many of the new "cough drop" products now contain pectin, rather than menthol. Pectin is a natural occurring product, which is obtained from the inner rind of citrus fruits and from apples. Pectin is considered a demulcent, a substance which is capable of soothing inflamed or abraded mucous membrane or protects it from irritation.

Above I mentioned alcoholic beverages and its effects on the throat and sinus infections. I found the same held true for mouthwashes or gargles that also contain alcohol. Now this doesn't mean that one has to stop using these products completely. *I RECOMMEND NOT USING THESE PRODUCTS WHEN YOU HAVE A SORE THROAT.* If you must use one, presently there are several companies that now produce a mouthwash and/or gargle that contain NO alcohol as one of its ingredients.

Let's take this a little further. We know that the natural occurring allicin in an ordinary raw fresh white onion can prevent the onset of a sore throat that can spread to the sinuses and ears, if used within a four- hour time frame of feeling the onset of a scratchy sore throat. But what was causing these infections? Yes, we know it's a bacterium that caused the infection, but what set me up for the infection? Sure, exposure to someone else who was infected was one way, or using contaminated drinking or eating utensils is another. In my case I wanted to know how, when, and why.

There were two or three times I was late with the "onion treatment" and my sore throats would spread into full- blown sinus infections. Like mentioned before the times were early spring and late fall.

Finally I figured it out. Each time it happened was right after I tried to catch a few rays of sunshine to start an early suntan in the early spring or in the late fall to enhance my tan.

Residing in Seattle gives one the advantage of enjoying the year's early and late sunshine to develop and maintain a suntan. Here you can lie in the sun when the temperature is in the low 60's without feeling cold, because there is usually little wind and not too much humidity. Now I wait till the temperature is at least 68° before attempting to soak up a few rays, and so far as I expected, I no longer have sore throats or sinus infections to fight. Thank Goodness!

After surveying people who asked my advice about sore throats and sinus and ear infections, I found that many who were struck with such infections were those who would completely turn off their heat in their homes at night or set the thermostat below 65°F. If you're having problems, watch this. Also, depending on the temperature outside, I highly recommend opening the bedroom window at least slightly, so you'll have fresh air to breathe during your sleeping hours.

If you begin to feel the start of a sore throat, chop up some fresh (it has to be fresh) peeled white onion, and serve it raw on a cooked hot dog. How much onion? About two teaspoonfuls will do. If you don't like or can't eat hot dogs, just eat the raw onions on some plain bread or just chew a bite or two of the sliced white onion and swirl the bite around your mouth for about 20 seconds and swallow. If doing so would be upsetting to your stomach, just swallow the created juices and spit out the remaining pulp. After the onion treatment be sure to wait about ten to fifteen minutes before eating or drinking any thing else. This gives the allicin in the onion time to sterilize your throat, sinuses, and ear passages. Caution should be taken with the "onion treatment." It should not be used by youngsters under six years of age, for the onions may be too strong to eat and usually more than four hours go by before you become aware of the malady in these young folks. If you have chronic sore throat, sinus, or ear infections, make the raw fresh white onion treatment part of your regular diet. Remember now ... use *moderation!*

There are some people who seldom have a cold, flu, sore throat or sinus infection. All I can say, as I have said before, is that outside of a natural immunity or of not being exposed, they most likely drink or eat grape juice, onions or other food products that unbeknownst to them keep them healthy.

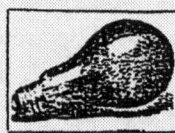

SIDE LITE

It was a 4th of July weekend, and I had just opened the pharmacy for business. No sooner had the doors opened, and there were four calls from dentists for their patients. Each call was for two prescriptions, one an antibiotic and the other pain pills. The dentists were all treating people with abscessed teeth. Right after the four phone calls, two walk- in patients also came to the pharmacy with the same two prescriptions medications for an abscessed tooth. Was this a coincidence or what? The pharmacy was a very high volume prescription location. After filling the prescriptions for the six individuals with abscess teeth, I figured there had to be some sort of pattern. It didn't take long to make some sense of the happening. Just like colds, flu, sore throats, and sinus infections, I noticed certain ills occurred around the same time, usually twice a year. They were more prevalent twice a year: however, the ills could affect people at lower levels any time throughout the year. The pharmacy would fill unusually greater amounts of prescriptions for asthma in January and August. For children we had the most prescriptions for ear infections in May and August. As mentioned earlier most throat and sinus infection took place in April and early May and again in October. Hemorrhoids cause their major problems in January and August. Oh, as far as abscessed teeth, the most prevalent time for such infections is the last week of June going into the first week of July and around the end of November and the beginning of December. Ulcer attacks are prominent in the spring and fall.

Migraine headaches most often flare up in late November and late February and the first week of March. Let me give you an example of how this information can assist you in preventing illness. It's known that certain foods can precipitate a migraine attack. Obviously, one should avoid certain foods that cause migraines, but even more so at times when attacks are most likely to occur. A young lady working in the same office where I was employed asked my advice about migraine attacks she was having. I told her what foods to avoid such attacks, and she had success in decreasing her number of migraine headaches. Months later while crossing paths in the office hallway, I reminded her to be especially careful for it was that time of the year for migraine headaches to be more prevalent. She told me she believed about the foods not to eat to prevent attacks, but as far as the thing about the time of year, she brushed that off. The next morning one the local newspaper's sport page headlined a story of a star player for the professional basketball team that didn't play the night before due to a migraine attack. Later in the day the young lady came up to my office. She told me she read the sport page headline and that she now believes.

What about colds and flu? What I have noticed is that both usually have two major outbreaks during the year with one of the two outbreaks more severe than the other. The two severe outbreaks most often occur between the middle of October and the end of April. As mentioned previously, both colds and flu can afflict anyone at anytime throughout the year.

The time frames mentioned are for the Seattle, WA area, and most likely may vary with geographical location and weather conditions.

Conclusion

As I MENTIONED in the Preface of this book and I believe it is worth repeating here again, prevention of disease is the medicine of the present time and the future. The focus on prevention will help people of all ages lead a longer, healthier, and more productive life. Billions and billions of health dollars can be saved. Take a second and just think about what great benefits those saved healthcare dollars could have and what good use these dollars could be put to in the world today. The same anti-viral concepts presented to you in this publication most likely can be utilized to prevent not only the common cold and flu, but who knows what other viral infections such as Epstein-Barr, SARS (Severe Acute Respiratory Syndrome), which is caused by a virus similar to the common cold virus, and the norovirus, a Norwalk-like virus which is causing havoc with the cruise ship industry… and last but not least, Bird Flu or the H5N1 virus.

Let me tell you, coming up with a new health concept or idea, of which I have many, can lead to some ridicule and "ribbing." Thank goodness mine was all in good fun. I made no secret of my prevention finds. I said previously I told my relatives, friends, neighbors, pharmacy patrons, and all those who would listen of the healthful properties of grapes and onions. Many times I would be greeted with, "Are you feeling 'grape' today? Or "I'm surprised you haven't turned purple yet with all the grape juice you drink." The ultimate "jest" came at a going away party given for me when changing employers. It was a fabulous party given for me by my peers. And guess how the celebration cake was decorated? In case you haven't, let me tell you. The main cake decorations were a bunch of grapes and a freshly peeled white onion.

As far as having to drink grape juice to prevent colds and flu or eat raw white onion to prevent sore throats that can also proceed into sinus and ear infections, after reading "THE J.ALBERT ANTIVIRAL RE-PORT", I'm sure a few pharmaceutical companies with all their modern research and technology will develop and market products based on what is presented in the report... maybe a sugarless chewing gum, a chewable candy, a troche, or a lozenge. Can you envision a sugarless antiviral chewable "gummi bear" candy? I know I can.

Oh, and before I forget, what about allicin products to prevent throat, sinus, and ear bacterial infections. Again, the products would be in an easy to use form.

May the antiviral information revealed in this book lead to further research that will rid mankind of the colds and flu forever.

NATURE HAS A SOLUTION FOR EVERY SITUATION. ALL ONE HAS TO DO IS DISCOVER IT.

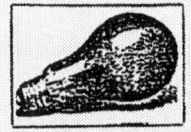

SIDE LITE

Recently I developed a heart condition. After doing a little research I found that the omega-3 in salmon can assist in treating this ailment. I never cared much for fish; however, salmon is now part of my regular diet. On my last visit to my cardiologist I mentioned to him that I have now eaten so much salmon that when I go for a dip in a river, I immediately start swimming upstream.

If you have a certain disease, illness, or sickness, I challenge you to do all you can to conquer the situation. As seen too often in my career as a pharmacist:

And as I said previously:

"GOOD HEALTH IS AN ASSET MANY DO NOT VALUE UNTIL THEY LOSE IT. AND AFTER ONCE LOST, TOO OFTEN NOT ALL THE MONEY IN THE WORLD CAN BUY IT BACK." TAKE CARE! VALUE AND CHERISH YOUR HEALTH.

"GOOD HEALTH TO YOU AND ALL THE WORLD"
—J. Albert

Now that you have spent your good money and time reading this book, use the information I have revealed to you, so you may lead a healthier more productive life. Share this information with your family, neighbors, friends, and fellow workers. Let's make the common cold and flu uncommon to all.

DURING THE WRITING OF THIS BOOK I BELIEVE I FIGURED OUT WHY I ACCOMPLISHED MUCH LESS AS I GET FURTHER INTO RETIREMENT. IT'S BECAUSE AS ONE GETS OLDER "TIME GOES FASTER."

"WITH RESEARCH ON THE COMMON COLD I SAW WHAT EVERYBODY ELSE SAW, AND THOUGHT WHAT NOBODY ELSE DID THINK."

—J. ALBERT HERMLE

EPILOGUE

HERE IT IS November 2006, and *FINALLY!!! STOP HAVING COLDS & FLU* is still not in publication! Till this time I never realized how hard it was to get a book into print.

ANOTHER CASE HISTORY…

Before I conclude, let me tell you of another very recent case history involving my antiviral findings.

It was late August or early September while making a transaction at my local credit union that I encountered a young account executive, who after discovering I was a pharmacist, asked what she could do to prevent her entire family from getting bouts of both colds and flu.

She told me her family, which included school children, were devastated with colds and flu the previous few years. With an opening like that and just as I most often have done in the past, I revealed to her my antiviral findings. She said my information sounded very natural and easy to do and she would have her whole family do it.

About a year and a half later in late January I encountered the young lady again while at the credit union. I asked if she had followed my antiviral revelations. She said the whole family did.

What were the results? For the past year and a half, there were NO colds or flu in her family! Also, she said she used my recommendation a few times to prevented throat infections. She did this by eating some fresh white peeled onion.

And last, but not least: for me it has been another year of NO colds or flu during the 2004 – 2007 cold & flu seasons! Oh, as far as throat, sinus, and ear infections go, I had none of those.

**IN THE INTEREST OF MY OWN ON-GOING PERSONAL
RESEARCH AND STUDY OF THE COMMON COLD
AND FLU, I HAVE NEVER HAD A FLU SHOT.
THAT'S RIGHT . . . NO FLU SHOT. SO FAR, SO GOOD!**

FINALLY!!! STOP HAVING COLDS & FLU "OUTTAKES"

The following are a few stories along with a little humor that I intended to use in this book. However, they were not used because I thought they didn't quite fit properly into the presentation.

I hope you enjoy.

Being a Director of Pharmacy for a large supermarket chain, I traveled many miles throughout Washington State to both hire pharmacists and open new pharmacies for the chain. I've said that I drove so many miles throughout the state *that when I got lost I knew exactly where I was.*

A friend of mine always gets the attention of various groups of golfers he meets for the first time by announcing he usually shoots in the 70's. Then as all ears perk up, and he has everyone's attention, he mentions that if it gets any warmer he doesn't play.

I opened two new pharmacy locations in the city of Walla Walla, Washington in the late 1990's. I always said that I opened one new pharmacy in this town for each Walla.

Father in Law: "Did you know that Joe is Magic?"
My Wife: "No, what do you mean?"
Father in Law: "Well, just the other day I saw Joe walking down the street, and he *"TURNED-INTO-A-DRUGSTORE."*

Patient: "Doctor, will I be able to play the piano after the operations on my hands?"
Doctor: "You sure will."
Patient: "That's just great! I never could before."

For 20 years my wife taught piano lessons while our three daughters were growing up. When the girls were old enough to be on their own, she went back to school to earn a degree in teaching followed by a Masters Degree in Education. She did this to get a position as a music teacher in the public schools. Currently she is well into her 25th year of teaching

Throughout her teaching career she developed many accomplished musicians. However, she seldom mentions or tells anyone of her great results of teaching music. I tell all that she is a music teacher who **"NEVER TOOTS HER OWN HORN."**

Because I lost so much hair over the years, I asked my barber for a discount on the haircut I was about to receive. He said that if he gave me a discount, he would have to charge me a "finder's fee", which would make the haircut more expensive.

As mentioned above I lost much of my hair over the years. Well, my grandson was visiting, and I told him I would have to get a hair cut later in the day. He said, "Not a hair cut Grandpa; you are going to get an "air" cut."

Sam: "What's an illusion?"
Joey: "An illusion is an optical conclusion."

Twice I was involved in an auto accident, and each time I bumped my head.

My mother always said son, when you get in trouble use your head.

Patient: "Doctor, it hurts when I do that!"
Doctor: "Well, don't do that."

All things come to an end. It's my wish that reading this book will be good for your health and life.

HEALTHY QUOTATIONS

It's easy to quit smoking. I quit when I was eleven.

-J. ALBERT

Health and intellect are the two blessings of life.

-MENANDER

The beginning of health is to know the disease.

-CERVANTES

A man to busy to take care of his health is like a mechanic too busy to take care of their tools.

-SPANISH PROVERB

To get rich never risk your health. For it is truth that health is the wealth of wealth.

-RICHARD BAKER

The greatest of follies is to sacrifice health for any other kind of happiness.

-ARTHUR SCHOPENHAUER

Happiness lies, first of all, in health.

-G.W.CURTIS

O health! health! The blessing of the rich! The riches of the poor! Who can buy thee at to dear a rate, since there is no enjoying this world without thee.

-Ben Johnson

Without health, life is not life; life is lifeless.

-ARIPHON THE SICYONIAN

He who hath good health is young.

-H. G. BOHN

Health is not valued till sickness comes.

-THOMAS FULLER

Diet cures more than doctors.

-A.B. CHEALES

In health there is freedom. Health is the first of all liberties.

-HENRI-FREDERIC AMIEL

The body is like a piano, and happiness is like music. It is needful to have the instrument in good order.

-BEECHER

Health is the vital principle of bliss, and exercise, of health.

-JAMES THOMSON

As I see it everyday you do one of two things: build health or produce disease in yourself.

-ADELE DAVIS

Sedentary people have shriveled hearts and most of us who do not exercise have an atrophied body.

-DR. BRUCE B. DAN

[Nature] can refuse to speak but she cannot give the wrong answer.

-DR. CHARLES HUGGINS

Health and good estate of body are above all gold, and a strong body above infinite wealth.

-APOCRYPHA ECCLESIASTICUS, xxx, 15

Health and an able body are two jewels.

-JOHN FLETCHER

The preservation of health is a duty, few seem conscious that there is such a thing as physical morality.

-HERBERT SPENCER

Take care of your body. It's the only place you have to live.

-JIM ROHM

Health is the thing that makes you feel that now is the best time of year.

-FRANKLIN P. ADAMS

Prevention is better than cure.

-PROVERB

We know a great deal more about the causes of physical disease than we do about the cause of physical health.

-M. SCOTT PECK

Jogging and exercise are like beating your head against a wall. You feel so good when you're finished.

-J. ALBERT

Guard your health.

-CICERO

HEALTH LOG

HEALTH LOG

Proper DIET, EXERCISE, and REST are three of many very important PILLARS OF HEALTH. Use each with their many subsets to maintain or improve your health.

<u>What are some of the subsets?</u>

**Under DIET there's weight, blood pressure, blood sugar, and calorie control.
Under EXERCISE there's jogging and running times, stretching and weight training.
Under REST there's sleep, nap, yoga, and meditation.
The above are just a few of the many subsets of the THREE PILLARS that a person may use to improve their health.**

Use the following three logs to list and track your own personal health goals and accomplishments, whatever they may be. You may customize the log pages to fit your own needs.

DIET NOTES

GOAL: _____

_____

ACTION PLAN: _____

_____

_____

STARTING DATE: _____
PROGRESS: _____

_____

_____

_____

_____

_____

_____

DATE GOAL MET: _____

DIET NOTES

GOAL: _____

_____

ACTION PLAN: _____

_____

_____

STARTING DATE: _____
PROGRESS: _____

_____

_____

_____

_____

_____

_____

DATE GOAL MET: _____

DIET NOTES

GOAL: _____

_____

_____

ACTION PLAN: _____

_____

_____

STARTING DATE: _____
PROGRESS: _____

_____

_____

_____

_____

_____

_____

_____

DATE GOAL MET: _____

EXERCISE NOTES

GOAL: _____

_____

ACTION PLAN: _____

_____

_____

STARTING DATE: _____
PROGRESS: _____

_____

_____

_____

_____

_____

_____

DATE GOAL MET: _____

EXERCISE NOTES

GOAL: _____

_____

ACTION PLAN: _____

_____

_____

STARTING DATE: _____
PROGRESS: _____

_____

_____

_____

_____

_____

_____

DATE GOAL MET: _____

EXERCISE NOTES

GOAL: _____

_____

_____

ACTION PLAN: _____

_____

_____

STARTING DATE: _____

PROGRESS: _____

_____

_____

_____

_____

_____

_____

_____

DATE GOAL MET: _____

REST NOTES

GOAL:_____
_____
_____

ACTION PLAN:_____
_____
_____
_____

STARTING DATE:_____
PROGRESS:_____
_____
_____
_____
_____
_____
_____
_____

DATE GOAL MET:_____

REST NOTES

GOAL: _____

_____

ACTION PLAN: _____

_____

_____

STARTING DATE: _____
PROGRESS: _____

_____

_____

_____

_____

_____

_____

DATE GOAL MET: _____

REST NOTES

GOAL: _____

_____

_____

ACTION PLAN: _____

_____

_____

STARTING DATE: _____
PROGRESS: _____

_____

_____

_____

_____

_____

_____

_____

DATE GOAL MET: _____

FOR SMOKERS ONLY...

NOW IS THE TIME TO MAKE THAT COMMITMENT TO STOP THE HABIT!!!

ACTION PLAN: _____

_____

_____

_____

STARTING DATE: _____
PROGRESS: _____

_____

_____

_____

_____

_____

DATE GOAL MET: _____

****

If all my patients were to follow J. Albert's antiviral cold and flu prevention program, my medical practice would decrease by about one third.

-A SEATTLE/TACOMA AREA, WA PHYSICIAN

****